FIBROMYALGIA COOKBOOK

MAIN COURSE – 80+ Fibromyalgia-friendly recipes for fast pain relief, reduce inflammation and faster physical recovery

TABLE OF CONTENTS

BREAKFAST 7
MUSHROOM OMELETTE 7
AVOCADO TOAST 8
TOMATO SHAKSHUKA 9
PORTOBELLO MUSHROOM CAPS 11
EGG IN AVOCADO 12
OMELETTE BITES 13
MACADAMIA WAFFLES 14
BACON & AVOCADO SANDWICHES 15
ZUCCHINI FRITTATA 16
SWEET POTATO BREAKFAST CAKE 18
MINI EGG OMELETS 19
BREAKFAST MEATCAKES 20
BROCCOLI FRITTATA 22
SWEET POTATO FRITTATA 23
BREAKFAST MEATLOAF 24
SALMON FRITATTA 26
BREAKFAST SAUSAGE SCOTCH EGGS 27
BREAKFAST COOKIES 28
PUMPKIN PANCAKES 30
SALMON FRITATTA 31
LUNCH 32
SPLIT PEA SOUP 32
CHICKEN SALAD 33
LENTIL PIE 35

CHICKEN SOUP	37
SLOW COOKER ZITI	38
LEMON GARLIC CHICKEN	40
BEEF STROGANOFF	41
PUMPKIN, CHILI AND COCONUT SOUP	43
KALE CAESAR SALAD	44
TILAPIA WITH PECAN ROSEMARY	45
ROASTED RED PEPPER SOUP	47
CHICKEN THIGHS WITH BRUSSELS SPROUTS AND POTATOES	48
CHICKEN STIR FRY	50
MEATBALLS	51
CHICKEN SALAD SLIDERS	52
CAULIFLOWER RICE	53
CAULIFLOWER MAC AND CHEESE	54
CHICKEN TENDERS	56
CHICKEN THIGHS WITH BUTTERNUT SQUASH	57
TACO LASAGNA	58
DINNER	60
HONEY SALMON	60
STUFFED SWEET POTATOES	61
MUSHROOM STROGANOFF	62
BLACK BEAN BURGERS	63
SPICED CHICKEN	65
OLIVE OIL & HERBS SALMON	67
LEMON CHICKEN THIGHS	68
GARLIC ZUCCHINI	69

RADISHES & ASPARAGUS WITH MINT	70
GINGER, BUTTERNUT SQUASH & SWEET POTATO	72
BREADED TURKEY	73
LENTILS	74
HUMMUS	75
BEANS BURGERS	76
BORLOTTI BEAN	77
FOIL COOKED FISH	79
GARLIC MUSHROOMS	80
TOFU BURGER	81
SWEET POTATOES FRIES	82
CHICKEN	83
SNACKS & DESSERTS	85
BLUEBERRY BAKED OATMEAL	85
OATMEAL COOKIE GRANOLA	86
HONEY WALNUTS	87
MUG CAKE	88
LEMON BITES	89
CHIA PUDDING	91
AVOCADO CAKE	92
APPLE COOKIES	93
PUMPKIN CHEESECAKE BARS	94
PUMPKIN CHEESECAKE	96
CELERY CARROT JUICE	98
SPINACH SMOOTHIE	99
KALE SMOOTHIE	100

STRAWBERRIES SMOOTHIE 101

PINEAPPLE SMOOTHIE 102

MANGO SALSA JUICE 103

GINGER JUICE 104

OATS SMOOTHIE 105

KIWI JUICE 106

PAIN KILLER JUICE 107

Copyright 2018 by Noah Jerris - All rights reserved.

This document is geared towards providing exact and reliable information in regards to the topic and issue covered. The publication is sold with the idea that the publisher is not required to render accounting, officially permitted, or otherwise, qualified services. If advice is necessary, legal or professional, a practiced individual in the profession should be ordered.

- From a Declaration of Principles which was accepted and approved equally by a Committee of the American Bar Association and a Committee of Publishers and Associations.

In no way is it legal to reproduce, duplicate, or transmit any part of this document in either electronic means or in printed format. Recording of this publication is strictly prohibited and any storage of this document is not allowed unless with written permission from the publisher. All rights reserved.

The information provided herein is stated to be truthful and consistent, in that any liability, in terms of inattention or otherwise, by any usage or abuse of any policies, processes, or directions contained within is the solitary and utter responsibility of the recipient reader. Under no circumstances will any legal responsibility or blame be held against the publisher for any reparation, damages, or monetary loss due to the information herein, either directly or indirectly.

Respective authors own all copyrights not held by the publisher.

The information herein is offered for informational purposes solely, and is universal as so. The presentation of the information is without contract or any type of guarantee assurance.

The trademarks that are used are without any consent, and the publication of the trademark is without permission or backing by the trademark owner. All trademarks and brands within this book are for clarifying purposes only and are the owned by the owners themselves, not affiliated with this document.

Introduction

Fibromyalgia recipes for personal enjoyment but also for family enjoyment. You will love them for sure for how easy it is to prepare them.

BREAKFAST

MUSHROOM OMELETTE

Serves: **1**

Prep Time: **5** Minutes

Cook Time: **5** Minutes

Total Time: **10** Minutes

INGREDIENTS

- 2 eggs
- Bacon
- 2 tsp coconut oil
- Nutmeg
- 1 red onion
- Salt
- Pepper

DIRECTIONS

1. Sauté the onion in the coconut oil for a few minutes.
2. Slice the mushrooms and add them to the pan, with salt and nutmeg.
3. Cook for another few minutes.

4. Remove the mushrooms from the pan.
5. Cook the beaten eggs for 3 minutes.
6. Serve the omelette topped with the mushroom mixture and bacon.

AVOCADO TOAST

Serves: *1*
Prep Time: *5* Minutes
Cook Time: *10* Minutes
Total Time: *15* Minutes

INGREDIENTS

- 1 clove garlic
- ½ avocado
- 1 egg
- Salt
- 1 slice toast
- Pepper
- Red pepper flakes

DIRECTIONS

1. Grate ½ clove of garlic into a pan, add the egg on top and cook to the desired degree of doneness.
2. Toast the bread.
3. Smash the avocado with a fork.
4. Spread the avocado over the toast.
5. Top with the fried egg and garlic, season, and serve.

TOMATO SHAKSHUKA

Serves: *4*

Prep Time: *10* Minutes

Cook Time: *50* Minutes

Total Time: *60* Minutes

INGREDIENTS

- 1 pinch cayenne
- Salt
- 1 red bell pepper
- 4 eggs
- ¼ cup olive oil

- 1 tbs cumin seeds
- 1 yellow onion
- 2 thyme sprigs
- 1 tbs parsley
- 1 ½ lb cherry tomatoes

DIRECTIONS

1. Preheat the oven to 350F.
2. Cut the tomatoes and place them on a cookie sheet, then season with salt.
3. Bake until fully roasted.
4. Roast the cumin seeds for 1 minute.
5. Add the olive oil and onion and saute until soft.
6. Add the strips chopped pepper, chopped herbs, and tomatoes.
7. Add the salt and cayenne pepper.
8. Pour the eggs into the pan and cook on low until the egg white is set.
9. Serve immediately.

PORTOBELLO MUSHROOM CAPS

Serves: **1**

Prep Time: **5** Minutes

Cook Time: **5** Minutes

Total Time: **10** Minutes

INGREDIENTS

- 50g ham
- Salt
- Pepper
- ¼ cup watercress
- 1 Portobello mushroom
- 1 poached egg
- ½ avocado

DIRECTIONS

1. Cook the mushrooms in coconut oil for 1 minute per side.
2. Season with salt and set aside.
3. Poach the eggs.
4. Pot each Portobello cap with the sliced avocado, a handful of watercress leaves, and ham.

5. Place the egg over, sprinkle with salt and pepper and serve.

EGG IN AVOCADO

Serves: 2
Prep Time: 5 Minutes
Cook Time: 10 Minutes
Total Time: 15 Minutes

INGREDIENTS

- 1 avocado
- 2 eggs
- Cheese
- Salt
- Pepper

DIRECTIONS

1. Preheat the oven to 425F.
2. Slice the avocado in half and remove the pit.
3. Crave out a little space in the center and crack the egg there.

4. Top with cheese.
5. Cook until the cheese is melted and the egg is done.
6. Serve immediately.

OMELETTE BITES

Serves: **12**

Prep Time: **5** Minutes

Cook Time: **35** Minutes

Total Time: **40** Minutes

INGREDIENTS

- 4 eggs
- 1 green pepper
- 2 cups diced cooked chicken
- 2 cups spinach
- 1 avocado
- 12 egg whites
- Pepper
- 12 slices bacon
- 1 red pepper

DIRECTIONS

1. Preheat the oven to 350F.
2. Cook the bacon for 5 minutes, making sure it's not crispy.
3. Grease a muffin tin and place one piece of bacon in each tin, wrapping it around the outer edges.
4. Whisk together in a bowl the eggs, egg whites, salt, pepper, peppers, chicken, and spinach.
5. Mix well then pour into each muffin tin.
6. Bake for 30 minutes, serve topped with avocado.

MACADAMIA WAFFLES

Serves: **6**

Prep Time: **10** Minutes

Cook Time: **3** Minutes

Total Time: **40** Minutes

INGREDIENTS

- 4 tbs coconut flour

- 1 cup macadamia nuts
- ½ cup coconut milk
- 1 tsp baking powder
- 3 eggs
- 1 tsp vanilla
- 3 tbs maple syrup
- 3 tbs coconut oil

DIRECTIONS

1. Preheat the waffle iron.
2. Blend all of the ingredients for 30 seconds on low.
3. Blend on high for another 30 seconds, until completely smooth.
4. Pour the batter into the waffle iron.
5. Cook on low for 50 seconds.
6. Serve topped with your desired syrups.

BACON & AVOCADO SANDWICHES

Serves: 2
Prep Time: 5 Minutes
Cook Time: 5 Minutes

Total Time: **10** Minutes

INGREDIENTS

- Salt
- 1 avocado
- 4 strips bacon
- 1 lime

DIRECTIONS

1. Cook the bacon.
2. Mash the avocado with lime juice and salt.
3. Place the avocado mixture between the bacon slices.
4. Serve immediately.

ZUCCHINI FRITTATA

Serves: **4**
Prep Time: **10** Minutes
Cook Time: **25** Minutes
Total Time: **35** Minutes

INGREDIENTS

- 1 sweet potato
- 2 zucchinis
- 8 eggs
- 1 red bell pepper
- 2 tbs coconut oil
- 2 tbs parsley
- Salt
- Pepper

DIRECTIONS

1. Cook the potato slices in the oil for 10 minutes.
2. Add the zucchini and bell peppers and cook for another 5 minutes.
3. Whisk the eggs in a bowl.
4. Season with salt and pepper and add it to the veggies.
5. Cook on low for 10 minutes.
6. Serve topped with fresh parsley.

SWEET POTATO BREAKFAST CAKE

Serves: **4**

Prep Time: **30** Minutes

Cook Time: **15** Minutes

Total Time: **35** Minutes

INGREDIENTS

- 2 tbs oil
- 2 tbs parsley
- 1 red onion
- 3 egg whites
- 2 sweet potatoes
- ½ cup dried cranberries
- 6 eggs
- Salt
- Pepper

DIRECTIONS

1. Preheat the oven to 425F.
2. Poke holes all around the potatoes using a fork.
3. Add the cranberries, parsley, onion, salt, and pepper.
4. Add 2 whisked egg whites.

5. Make patties from the mixture.
6. Cook in oil for 4 minutes on each side.
7. Place the cooked patties onto a greased baking dish.
8. Push down in the middle of each patty, creating space for the eggs.
9. Crack the eggs on top, into the created space.
10. Bake for 15 minutes.
11. Caramelize the onion in a skillet.
12. Serve topped with the caramelized onions.

MINI EGG OMELETS

Serves: **4**

Prep Time: **10** Minutes

Cook Time: **20** Minutes

Total Time: **30** Minutes

INGREDIENTS

- ¼ cup shredded cheddar
- 4 eggs
- ¼ cup cheese

- 1 ½ tsp olive oil
- 4 cups broccoli florets
- Salt
- Pepper
- 1 cup egg whites

DIRECTIONS

1. Preheat the oven to 350F.
2. Steam the broccoli for 5 minutes.
3. Once cooked, crumble into smaller pieces and add olive oil, salt, and pepper.
4. Grease a muffin tin and pour the mixture into each tin.
5. Beat the egg whites, eggs, cheese, salt and pepper in a bowl.
6. Pour over the broccoli, top with cheese and cook for 20 minutes.

BREAKFAST MEATCAKES

Serves: **14**

Prep Time: **10** Minutes

Cook Time: **40** Minutes

Total Time: **50** Minutes

INGREDIENTS

- 1 lb pork sausage
- 6 ounces blackberries
- 1 tsp cinnamon
- 1 ½ tsp salt
- 1 tsp black pepper
- 1 tsp rosemary
- 1 tsp thyme
- 1 orange zest
- 1 ln chicken breast
- 12 strips bacon
- 1 apple
- 1 tsp garlic powder

DIRECTIONS

1. Preheat the oven to 375F.
2. Dice the apple.
3. Line the cupcake pans with bacon.
4. Mix together, smashing with hands, sausage, spices, chicken, apple, zest, and blackberries.
5. Fill the pan with the mixture.
6. Bake for 35 minutes.
7. Serve topped with zest or blackberries.

BROCCOLI FRITTATA

Serves: **8**

Prep Time: **10** Minutes

Cook Time: **3** Minutes

Total Time: **40** Minutes

INGREDIENTS

- 4 cups broccoli florets
- ½ tsp oregano
- 4 cups spinach
- 2 tbs coconut oil
- 1 onion
- 1 tsp salt
- 8 eggs
- 4 cloves garlic

DIRECTIONS

1. Preheat the oven to 350F.
2. Steam broccoli for about 3 minutes.
3. Rinse with cold water and set aside.
4. Saute the onions in the coconut oil for 20 minutes.
5. Add the garlic and saute for another 2 minutes.

6. Add the spinach and season with salt.
7. Allow spinach to wilt.
8. Add rinsed broccoli, oregano and the rest of the salt.
9. Stir well to combine, then remove from heat.
10. Pour the eggs over the vegetables and bake for 20 minutes and 350F, serve immediately.

SWEET POTATO FRITTATA

Serves: 4
Prep Time: 15 Minutes
Cook Time: 40 Minutes
Total Time: 55 Minutes

INGREDIENTS

- 1 1-lb sweet potato
- ½ bunch green onions
- 8 eggs
- 2 slices of bacon

DIRECTIONS

1. Preheat the oven to 400F.
2. Cook the bacon until crispy.
3. Cut the sweet potato lengthwise, then into rounds.
4. Coat the pan with olive oil.
5. Place the sweet potato slices in the pan and cook for 10 minutes.
6. Whip the eggs, then pour over the sweet potatoes.
7. Return to oven and cook for another 30 minutes.
8. Cook the green onions for a few minutes in the bacon skillet, after removing the bacon and pouring the grease out.
9. Serve topped with the bacon and green onion.

BREAKFAST MEATLOAF

Serves: 4
Prep Time: 10 Minutes
Cook Time: 3 Hours
Total Time: 3h 10 Minutes

INGREDIENTS

- 1 tbs coconut oil

- 2 tsp fennel seeds
- 3 tsp oregano
- 1 ½ red pepper flakes
- 2 ½ tsp sage
- 2 cups diced onion
- 3 tsp thyme
- ½ cup almond flour
- 2 tbs maple syrup
- 1 tbs garlic powder
- 1 ½ tsp black pepper
- 1 tsp paprika
- 2 tsp salt
- 2 lbs ground pork
- 2 eggs

DIRECTIONS

1. Cook the onions in the coconut oil until soft and translucent.
2. Whisk all of the ingredients, except the ground pork to a bowl.
3. Add the ground pork and onions and mix well with your hands.
4. Place the mixture in the middle of the slow cooker.
5. Pat the top and put the lid on the slow cooker.
6. Cook on low for 3 hours.
7. Allow to sit for 15 minutes in the turned off slow cooker, then transfer it to another dish.
8. Serve immediately.

SALMON FRITATTA

Serves: **2**

Prep Time: **10** Minutes

Cook Time: **15** Minutes

Total Time: **25** Minutes

INGREDIENTS

- 6 eggs
- ½ onion
- ½ cup coconut milk
- ½ cup salmon
- 2 ½ tbs cilantro
- 2 garlic cloves
- 1 ½ cups cherry tomatoes
- 1 tsp cumin
- 1 tbs coconut oil
- 1 green pepper
- 1 tsp paprika
- Salt
- Pepper

DIRECTIONS

1. Preheat the oven to 350F.
2. Cook the green pepper and onion in the coconut oil, then add the garlic, cumin, paprika, salt, and pepper and allow to cook a little.
3. Add the halved tomatoes and allow to cook a bit.
4. Sprinkle in the salmon.
5. Mix the eggs and cream together, then pour the mixture in.
6. Season with salt and pepper.
7. Transfer to the oven and cook for 15 minutes.
8. Serve topped with fresh cilantro.

BREAKFAST SAUSAGE SCOTCH EGGS

Serves: 6
Prep Time: 25 Minutes
Cook Time: 25 Minutes
Total Time: 50 Minutes

INGREDIENTS

- 6 eggs
- 1 lb ground pork

- Cloves
- 1 ½ tsp cinnamon
- 1 tsp salt
- ½ tsp black pepper
- Nutmeg

DIRECTIONS

1. Cook the eggs by boiling them.
2. Preheat the oven to 350F.
3. Mix the ground pork, salt, pepper, and cinnamon until combined.
4. Cover the eggs with the meat mixture, creating an "armor".
5. Bake for 15 minutes, serve hot or cold.

BREAKFAST COOKIES

Serves: *12*
Prep Time: *10* Minutes
Cook Time: *15* Minutes
Total Time: *25* Minutes

INGREDIENTS

- ½ tsp salt
- 1 tsp baking soda
- ½ cup applesauce
- 2 eggs
- ½ tbs cinnamon
- 2 tbs dark cherries
- 2 ½ tbs walnuts
- ¼ cup coconut flour
- ½ cup almond butter
- 6 dried dates
- 1 cup shredded coconut
- 3 tbs currants
- 1 tsp vanilla

DIRECTIONS

1. Preheat the oven to 350F.
2. Process the coconut flour, dates, almond butter in a food processor.
3. Add the applesauce, cinnamon, coconut, eggs, vanilla, salt, and baking soda and process for another 30 seconds.
4. Add the remaining ingredients and pulse one more time.
5. Form balls from the dough and place them on a cookie sheet lined with parchment paper.
6. Bake for 15 minutes, then serve immediately.

PUMPKIN PANCAKES

Serves: **6**
Prep Time: **10**   Minutes
Cook Time: **20**   Minutes
Total Time: **30**   Minutes

INGREDIENTS

- 4 eggs
- ½ cup almond butter
- 2 tbs coconut oil
- ½ cup pumpkin puree
- 1 tsp vanilla
- ¼ cup coconut flour
- ¼ cup almond milk
- 1 tsp nutmeg
- ½ tsp ginger
- ½ tsp cardamom
- 1 tsp baking powder
- 2 tsp cinnamon
- ½ cup honey
- ½ tsp salt

DIRECTIONS

1. Preheat a greased pan.
2. Beat all of the wet ingredients together in a bowl.
3. Add the dry ingredients and beat until smooth.
4. Cook the pancakes for 30 seconds per side.
5. Serve topped with bacon, pecans, and maple syrup.

SALMON FRITATTA

Serves: **4**

Prep Time: **10** Minutes

Cook Time: **10** Minutes

Total Time: **20** Minutes

INGREDIENTS

- ½ tsp coconut oil
- 4 eggs
- 4 ounces salmon

DIRECTIONS

1. Add the beaten eggs into a well coated preheated pan.
2. Cook the eggs for about 5 minutes.
3. Place the pan into the broiler and cook until the eggs are done.
4. Remove from the broiler and allow to cool.
5. Serve topped with salmon.

LUNCH

SPLIT PEA SOUP

Serves: **8**

Prep Time: **10** Minutes

Cook Time: **4** Hours

Total Time: **4h 10** Minutes

INGREDIENTS

- 2 tsp cumin
- 2 cubes bouillon
- 2 potatoes
- 2 tsp sage
- 2 cups green split peas
- 1 ½ tsp thyme

- 3-4 bay leaves
- 3 carrots
- 1 onion
- 8 cups vegetable broth
- 3 cloves garlic
- 1 ½ tsp mustard

DIRECTIONS
1. Place the vegetable broth, split peas, and bouillon cubes into a slow cooker, then give it a good stir.
2. Add the celery, carrots, onion, chopped potatoes, and garlic.
3. Add the cumin, mustard, thyme, sage, and bay leaves.
4. Season with salt and pepper and stir well.
5. Cover and cook for 4 hours on low, remove the bay leaves, then serve.

CHICKEN SALAD

Serves: *1*
Prep Time: *15* Minutes
Cook Time: *20* Minutes
Total Time: *35* Minutes

INGREDIENTS

- 2 tbs olive oil
- 1 ½ tbs mayonnaise
- ½ tsp oregano
- 5 tbs red onion
- 1/3 cup cherry tomatoes
- ½ cup cucumber
- 1 ½ tbs Greek yogurt
- 3 tbs lemon juice
- 1 ½ pitas
- ¼ tsp cumin
- 1/8 tsp pepper
- 2 ounces chicken
- 1 cup parsley
- ½ tsp paprika

DIRECTIONS

1. Preheat the oven to 400F.
2. Cut the pita into wedges and place onto a baking sheet.
3. Mix the paprika, oregano, and cumin in a bowl.
4. Season the pita with the mixture.
5. Bake for 10 minutes.
6. Mix 2 tbs of red onion, mayonnaise, Greek yogurt, 1 tbs lemon juice, black pepper, and the rotisserie chicken.

7. Mix the parsley, tomatoes, cucumber, red onion, 2 tbs lemon juice, and olive oil.
8. Mix the ingredients, then top with the chicken salad and add the pita chips.

LENTIL PIE

Serves: **6**

Prep Time: **20** Minutes

Cook Time: **120** Minutes

Total Time: **140** Minutes

INGREDIENTS

- 250g green lentils
- 1 tsp cumin powder
- 1 carrot
- ¼ pumpkin
- 10 mushrooms
- 2 tsp tamari sauce
- 4 cups water
- 140g tomato paste
- 2 bay leaves

- 1 cup green peas
- 3 tomatoes
- 1 leek
- 1 brown onion
- 1 celery stalk
- 1 garlic clove
- Bragg seasoning
- 1 red chili
- 2 tbs olive oil

DIRECTIONS

1. Soak the lentils in 4 cups water and a pinch of salt overnight.
2. Boil water and simmer the lentils for 20 minutes.
3. Peel and chop onion, garlic and leek.
4. Heat the oil over low heat.
5. Saute the garlic, onion, turmeric, salt, pepper, leek, bragg seasoning, cumin for 15 minutes.
6. Add the pumpkin, and saute for another 15 minutes.
7. Add the remaining ingredients, and stir for another 15 minutes.
8. Add ¼ cup of water, lentils, bay leaves and simmer for 1 hour.
9. Season, remove the bay leaves and pour into dishes.
10. Grill for 20 minutes.
11. Serve garnished with parsley.

CHICKEN SOUP

Serves: *4*

Prep Time: *25* Minutes

Cook Time: *8* Hours

Total Time: *8h 25* Minutes

INGREDIENTS

- 1 ½ tsp oregano
- 1 tsp cumin
- Black pepper
- Salt
- 2 yellow squash
- 3 ounces green beans
- 1 ½ lb chicken thighs
- 1 tbs lime juice
- 3 tbs cilantro
- 2 cups chicken stock
- 1 can diced tomatoes
- 1 onion
- 1 can tomato sauce
- 1 can green chiles
- 1 tsp chili powder

- 1 bell pepper
- 1 garlic clove

DIRECTIONS

1. Mix the onion, diced tomatoes, chili powder, chicken, chicken stock, chiles, oregano, cumin, bell pepper, garlic, and diced tomatoes in a slow cooker.
2. Season and cook on low for 8 hours.
3. Add the squash and green beans and cook for another 30 minutes.
4. Stir in the lime juice and cilantro.
5. Serve garnished with cilantro.

SLOW COOKER ZITI

Serves: *8*

Prep Time: *20* Minutes

Cook Time: *4* Hours

Total Time: *4h 20* Minutes

INGREDIENTS

- 28 ounces can tomatoes
- 1 onion
- 1 tsp garlic
- 650 ml jar pasta sauce
- 2 ½ cups water
- 375 gram box Ziti
- 1 cup cheese
- 1 lb beef
- 1 tsp salt
- 1 tsp basil
- 1 tsp parsley

DIRECTIONS

1. Cook the beef and onion until browned.
2. Stir in the garlic and salt for 1 minute.
3. Add basil, pasta sauce, beef mixture, tomatoes, parsley, and water to a slow cooker, and stir.
4. Cook for 4 minutes.
5. Add the pasta and stir.
6. Cook covered for 30 minutes.
7. Sprinkle with cheese and cook for 5 minutes.

LEMON GARLIC CHICKEN

Serves: **6**

Prep Time: **25** Minutes

Cook Time: **4** Hours

Total Time: **4h 25** Minutes

INGREDIENTS

- 2 lbs red potatoes
- Salt
- Pepper
- 1 lb carrots
- 6 chicken thighs
- ¼ cup olive oil
- 3 tbs lemon juice
- 4 cloves garlic
- 1 lemon
- 1 sweet yellow onion
- 3 sprigs rosemary
- 6 sprigs thyme

DIRECTIONS

1. Place the onions, potatoes, carrots in a slow cooker.

2. Season, then stir in 2 cloves of garlic and half of the herbs.
3. Season the chicken and add them to the slow cooker.
4. Pour the olive oil over, lemon juice, herbs and the remaining garlic.
5. Cook for 8 hours.
6. Remove the chicken and broil for 5 minutes.
7. Serve with the vegetables.

BEEF STROGANOFF

Serves: 4
Prep Time: 20 Minutes
Cook Time: 4 Hours
Total Time: *4h 20* Minutes

INGREDIENTS

- 12 ounces pasta noodles
- 2 tbs garlic
- 1 tbs mustard
- 1 cup sour cream

- 2 cups beef broth
- 2 lb stew meat
- 1 cup mushrooms
- 3 tbs Worcestershire sauce
- 5 ounces cream cheese
- 5 tbs corn starch
- 2 ½ tsp seasoning
- Salt
- Pepper

DIRECTIONS

1. Grease the slow cooker, then add the meat and season with the seasoning, salt, and pepper.
2. Add the beef broth, garlic, mushrooms, mustard, and Worcestershire sauce.
3. Cook on high for 4 hours.
4. Stir in the cornstarch into ½ cup beef broth and add to the cooker 30 minutes before serving.
5. Add the sour cream and cheese cream and cook for another 30 minutes.
6. Stir in the noodles, and serve immediately garnished with thyme.

PUMPKIN, CHILI AND COCONUT SOUP

Serves: **4**

Prep Time: **15** Minutes

Cook Time: **30** Minutes

Total Time: **45** Minutes

INGREDIENTS

- 1 red chilli
- 1 carrot
- 1 tsp ginger
- 1 can coconut cream
- 1 ½ kg pumpkin
- 1 tbs vegetable oil
- 4 cups vegetable stock

DIRECTIONS

1. Cut the peeled carrot and pumpkin.
2. Heat 1 tbs oil in a pot.
3. Add the pumpkin and carrot and cook for 5 minutes.
4. Add 4 cups of stock, ginger and chopped chili.
5. Simmer for 20 minutes.
6. Remove from heat and blend.

7. Mix in the coconut cream and heat until it comes back to the boil, serve with croutons.

KALE CAESAR SALAD

Serves: 2
Prep Time: 10 Minutes
Cook Time: 0 Minutes
Total Time: 10 Minutes

INGREDIENTS

- 2 tortillas
- 1 cup cherry tomatoes
- 1 cup cheese
- 6 cups kale
- 1/8 cup olive oil
- Salt
- Pepper
- ½ coddled egg
- 8 ounces grilled chicken
- 1 clove garlic
- 1 tsp mustard

- 1 tsp honey
- 1/8 cup lemon juice

DIRECTIONS

1. Mix the egg, minced garlic, honey, olive oil, lemon juice, and mustard.
2. Whisk well, then season.
3. Add the chicken, kale, tomatoes and toss to coat with the dressing.
4. Add ¼ cup cheese.
5. Distribute the salad over the tortillas and sprinkle with ¼ cup of cheese.
6. Roll up the wraps, and serve immediately.

TILAPIA WITH PECAN ROSEMARY

Serves: **4**
Prep Time: **20** Minutes
Cook Time: **20** Minutes
Total Time: **40** Minutes

INGREDIENTS

- Cayenne pepper
- 1/3 cup breadcrumbs
- 2 tsp rosemary
- 1 ½ tsp olive oil
- 1 egg white
- 1/3 cup pecans
- 4 tilapia fillets
- ½ tsp brown sugar
- 1/8 tsp salt

DIRECTIONS

1. Preheat the oven to 350F.
2. Stir together the sugar, cayenne pepper, rosemary, pecans, breadcrumbs, and salt.
3. Add the olive oil and toss.
4. Bake for 10 minutes.
5. Whisk the egg white in a bowl and dip the fish into it then into the pecan mixture.
6. Bake for 10 minutes.
7. Serve immediately.

ROASTED RED PEPPER SOUP

Serves: **6**

Prep Time: **30** Minutes

Cook Time: **30** Minutes

Total Time: **60** Minutes

INGREDIENTS

- 4 cups vegetable broth
- 1 can green chiles
- 2 tsp cumin
- 2 tbs fresh cilantro
- 1 tbs lemon juice
- 4 ounces cream cheese
- 2 tbs olive oil
- 2 onions
- 1 jar roasted red peppers
- 2 tsp salt
- 1 tsp coriander
- 4 cups sweet potatoes

DIRECTIONS

1. Heat the oil in a pan.

2. Cook the onions until soft, then add the peppers, green chiles, coriander, cumin, and salt and cook for 3 minutes.
3. Stir in the roasted peppers juice, peeled and cubed potatoes, and the vegetable broth.
4. Bring to a boil, then reduce the heat and cook for 15 minutes.
5. Stir in the lemon juice and cilantro.
6. Blend half of the soup with the cream cheese, then add back into the soup, serve immediately.

CHICKEN THIGHS WITH BRUSSELS SPROUTS AND POTATOES

Serves: 4
Prep Time: 15 Minutes
Cook Time: 30 Minutes
Total Time: 45 Minutes

INGREDIENTS

- 2 tsp salt
- 1 tsp thyme
- 1 lb chicken thighs

- 1 lb potatoes
- 3 tbs olive oil
- 1 lemon
- 1 orange
- 1 tsp black pepper
- 2 cloves garlic
- 4 shallots
- 1 ½ tbs paprika
- 2 lb Brussels sprouts

DIRECTIONS

1. Preheat the oven to 450F.
2. Toss the Brussels sprouts, potatoes, shallots, lemon and orange slices with 1 tbs oil, 1 tsp salt, and ½ tsp pepper.
3. Pour into a baking dish.
4. Mix the garlic, remaining salt and pepper, thyme, lemon and orange zest, paprika, and 2 tsp oil in a bowl.
5. Toss the chicken into the mixture.
6. Place the chicken over the Brussels sprouts.
7. Roast for 25 minutes, then serve.

CHICKEN STIR FRY

Serves: **2**

Prep Time: **10** Minutes

Cook Time: **10** Minutes

Total Time: **20** Minutes

INGREDIENTS

- 2 bell peppers
- 2 chicken breasts
- 1 tsp cumin
- 1 tsp cayenne pepper
- 1 tsp olive oil
- ½ tsp paprika
- 2 cups broccoli florets

DIRECTIONS

1. Heat the oil in a pan.
2. Add the diced chicken and cook until browned.
3. Add the broccoli and peppers and cook for 5-10 minutes.
4. Add the spices and a little water.
5. Cook for another few minutes.

MEATBALLS

Serves: 8
Prep Time: 15 Minutes
Cook Time: 20 Minutes
Total Time: 35 Minutes

INGREDIENTS

- 3 tbs ketchup
- ½ cup breadcrumbs
- 2 garlic cloves
- 2 tsp salt
- 1 lb ground beef
- ½ cup onion
- 1 tsp pepper
- 1 ½ tbs parsley
- 1 egg
- ½ cup cheese

DIRECTIONS

1. Preheat the oven to 400F.
2. Mix all of the ingredients in a bowl.
3. Form balls and place them on a greased cookie sheet.

4. Cook for 20 minutes, allow to cool, then serve.

CHICKEN SALAD SLIDERS

Serves: **4**

Prep Time: **10** Minutes

Cook Time: **0** Minutes

Total Time: **10** Minutes

INGREDIENTS

- ¼ cup almonds
- 1 cup apples
- ¼ cup dried cranberries
- 1 tsp salt
- 4 buns
- ½ lb shredded rotisserie chicken
- ¾ cup Greek yogurt
- 1 cup grapes

DIRECTIONS

1. Combine all of the ingredients in a bowl, except the buns.
2. Place the mixture onto the buns and secure with a toothpick, serve immediately.

CAULIFLOWER RICE

Serves: **4**

Prep Time: **10** Minutes

Cook Time: **20** Minutes

Total Time: **30** Minutes

INGREDIENTS

- 2 tbs soy sauce
- ½ tsp sesame oil
- ½ onion
- 2 cloves garlic
- 1 cup carrots
- 1 tsp black pepper
- 1 cauliflower
- 1 egg
- 2 Tbs oil

- 2 green onions
- 2 tsp salt
- 1 cup peas

DIRECTIONS

1. Mince the cauliflower.
2. Cook the onion and garlic in the oil in a pan.
3. Add the cauliflower and sauté.
4. Add the peas and carrots and stir until combined.
5. Add the sesame oil, soy sauce, beaten egg, and black pepper.
6. Stir until well cooked.
7. Add green onions, season, stir and serve.

CAULIFLOWER MAC AND CHEESE

Serves: **6**
Prep Time: **20**   Minutes
Cook Time: **30**   Minutes
Total Time: **50**   Minutes

INGREDIENTS

- 1 tsp chives
- ½ cup coconut milk
- ½ cup yeast
- ½ lb bacon
- 2 heads cauliflower
- 1 tsp salt
- ½ tsp black pepper

DIRECTIONS

1. Cook the bacon until crispy.
2. Cut the cauliflower florets away from the stems.
3. Steam it in a bowl with ¼ cup water in the microwave for 5 minutes.
4. Transfer to the pot used to cook the bacon.
5. Add the remaining ingredients and stir, reserving half of the bacon and the chives for garnish.

CHICKEN TENDERS

Serves: **7**

Prep Time: **5** Minutes

Cook Time: **10** Minutes

Total Time: **15** Minutes

INGREDIENTS

- 1 tbs coconut milk
- 1 tsp salt
- ½ tsp black pepper
- 1 tsp garlic powder
- 1 ½ lb chicken
- 1 1/3 cups flour
- ½ tsp onion powder
- 2 eggs

DIRECTIONS

1. Preheat the oven to 425F.
2. Put the flour on a dish.
3. Whisk the eggs and mix with the milk in a bowl.
4. Mix the seasonings together.

5. Dip the chicken strips into the flour, egg mixture, and seasonings in this order.
6. Place onto a lined sheet tray.
7. Bake for 10 minutes, flipping over after 5 minutes.

CHICKEN THIGHS WITH BUTTERNUT SQUASH

Serves: 6
Prep Time: 20 Minutes
Cook Time: 30 Minutes
Total Time: 50 Minutes

INGREDIENTS

- ½ lb bacon
- Pepper
- 3 cup Butternut Squash
- 2 tbs oil
- 6 chicken thighs
- Sage
- Salt

DIRECTIONS

1. Preheat the oven to 425F.
2. Fry the bacon until crispy.
3. Sauté the butternut squash in the bacon grease.
4. Season and cook until soft, then remove.
5. Cook the chicken thighs for 10 minutes.
6. Flip the thighs over and add the butternut all around.
7. Place the skillet in the oven.
8. Bake for 15 minutes.
9. Serve topped with the bacon and sage.

TACO LASAGNA

Serves: **9**

Prep Time: **20** Minutes

Cook Time: **30** Minutes

Total Time: **50** Minutes

INGREDIENTS

- 3 cup cheese
- 2/3 cup water
- 1 can tomatoes
- ½ cup green pepper
- 1 lb ground beef
- taco seasoning
- 1 can black beans
- ½ cup chopped onion
- 6 tortillas
- 1 can refried beans

DIRECTIONS

1. Cook the beef, onion, and pepper over medium heat.
2. Add the taco seasoning and water and bring to a boil.
3. Stir in the tomatoes and black beans.
4. Simmer for 10 minutes.
5. Place 2 tortillas into a baking dish and spread half of the mixture over.
6. Sprinkle 1 cup cheese and repeat layers.
7. Top with cheese.
8. Cook until the cheese it melted for about 30 minutes.
9. Serve immediately.

DINNER

HONEY SALMON

Serves: 2
Prep Time: 10 Minutes
Cook Time: 10 Minutes
Total Time: 20 Minutes

INGREDIENTS

- 2 tbs honey
- 1 ½ tbs mustard
- 8 ounces salmon
- 2 tbs lemon juice
- Salt
- Pepper

DIRECTIONS

1. Preheat the oven to broil.
2. Mix the honey, lemon juice and mustard in a bowl.
3. Line a cooking sheet with foil.
4. Spread the mixture over the salmon.
5. Broil for 5 minutes on each side.

STUFFED SWEET POTATOES

Serves: **8**

Prep Time: **10** Minutes

Cook Time: **1** Hour

Total Time: **1h 10** Minutes

INGREDIENTS

- 2 ½ tbs milk
- 1 cup cheese
- ½ onion
- 1 cup broccoli
- 1 sweet potatoes
- 1 ½ tbs butter
- ½ cup sour cream

DIRECTIONS

1. Preheat the oven to 350F.
2. Bake the potatoes for 40 minutes.
3. Cut in half and allow to cool.
4. Saute the onion, garlic, and broccoli in the butter for 5 minutes.

5. Scoop out the sweet potato and mix with milk, sour cream and broccoli mixture.
6. Fill the potato skin with the mixture and top with the cheese.
7. Bake until cheese is melted and serve immediately.

MUSHROOM STROGANOFF

Serves: 2
Prep Time: 10 Minutes
Cook Time: 20 Minutes
Total Time: 30 Minutes

INGREDIENTS

- ½ tsp salt
- ½ cup vegetable broth
- ½ cup wine
- 1 ½ tbs thyme
- ½ cup green onions
- 1 garlic clove
- 2 tsp oil

- 1 cup mushrooms
- ½ tsp pepper
- ½ cup rice
- ½ cup sour cream

DIRECTIONS

1. Sauté the mushrooms in the oil for 5 minutes.
2. Add the garlic and the green onions and cook for another minute.
3. Add the rest of the ingredients except for the rice and sour cream.
4. Bring to a boil, then add the rice and stir.
5. Reduce the heat to low and cook for 15 minutes.
6. Stir in the sour cream.
7. Serve garnished with green onions.

BLACK BEAN BURGERS

Serves: 5
Prep Time: 15 Minutes
Cook Time: 30 Minutes

Total Time: 45   Minutes

INGREDIENTS

- ½ bell pepper
- 5 tbs flax
- ½ cup flour
- salt
- 3 cups black beans
- ½ tsp cinnamon
- 1 ½ tsp cumin
- 1 ½ tsp coriander
- 2 cups mushrooms
- 1 ½ tsp paprika
- 1 green onion
- ¾ cup corn
- ½ onion
- ½ cup cilantro
- 1 clove garlic
- 2 tsp oil

DIRECTIONS

1. Puree the mushrooms, onion, cilantro, and garlic.
2. Cook the mushroom mixture in the oil, adding the cinnamon, cumin, coriander and paprika for 5 minutes.
3. Add the diced peppers and cook for another minute.

4. Transfer the mixture in a bowl and mix in the beans, corn, green onion and flax meal.
5. Season with salt.
6. Shape the mixture into patties and cook for 5 minutes, then place in the oven for 10 minutes at 370F.
7. Serve on bun topped with your favorite toppings.

SPICED CHICKEN

Serves: **6**

Prep Time: **10** Minutes

Cook Time: **25** Minutes

Total Time: **35** Minutes

INGREDIENTS

- 1 cup pecans
- 1 ½ cups milk
- 1 tsp salt
- 4 chicken breasts
- 2 ½ tsp cumin
- 4 tbs oil
- 1 ½ tbs apple vinegar

- 1 tbs arrowroot starch
- 2 tbs water
- 1 tsp cinnamon
- Salt
- 1 clove garlic
- 2 apples
- 1 tsp cardamom

DIRECTIONS

1. Heat a skillet.
2. Pound the chicken breasts.
3. Stir together the cinnamon, cumin, salt and cardamom and coat the chicken with spices.
4. Cook the chicken in 2 tbs oil for 3 minutes until almost cooked, then remove from the pan.
5. Add the remaining oil, garlic, diced apples and pecans to the pan.
6. Cook for another 5 minutes.
7. Pour in the milk and vinegar.
8. Add the chicken.
9. Mix the arrowroot starch and water and pour into the pan.
10. Cook covered for 5 minutes.
11. Serve immediately.

OLIVE OIL & HERBS SALMON

Serves: **4**

Prep Time: **15** Minutes

Cook Time: **40** Minutes

Total Time: **55** Minutes

INGREDIENTS

- ½ cup oil
- 1 ½ lb salmon
- ¼ cup dill fronds
- ¼ cup tarragon leaves
- 1 lemon zest
- 1 shallot
- Salt
- Pepper

DIRECTIONS

1. Preheat the oven to 250F.
2. Cook the salmon in the oil in a large pan.
3. Process the dill, lemon zest, shallot and tarragon in a food processor.

4. Blend in 2 tbs of oil and pour the paste over the salmon.
5. Bake for 30 minutes and serve with green salad.

LEMON CHICKEN THIGHS

Serves: **4**

Prep Time: **10** Minutes

Cook Time: **30** Minutes

Total Time: **40** Minutes

INGREDIENTS

- 5 thyme sprigs
- Salt
- Pepper
- 2 lb chicken thighs
- Oil
- 1 lemon

DIRECTIONS

1. Preheat the oven to 400F.

2. Drizzle oil over the chicken and season with salt and pepper.
3. Cook over medium heat for 15 minutes.
4. When crispy, flip over and scatter lemon slices and thyme over.
5. Roast for another 15 minutes.
6. Serve immediately.

GARLIC ZUCCHINI

Serves: 4
Prep Time: 20 Minutes
Cook Time: 30 Minutes
Total Time: 50 Minutes

INGREDIENTS

- 3 tbs basil
- 1/3 cup oil
- ¼ cup red wine vinegar
- 2 lb zucchini
- Salt
- Pepper

- ¼ cup parsley
- 3 cloves garlic

DIRECTIONS

1. Sprinkle the zucchini with salt, let stand for 30 minutes, then rinse.
2. Mix the basil, parsley, and garlic in a bowl.
3. Fry the zucchini in the oil for about 5 minutes.
4. Transfer the zucchini to a plate and top with the herb mixture and the vinegar.
5. Season with salt and pepper.
6. Allow to cool, then serve.

RADISHES & ASPARAGUS WITH MINT

Serves: *4*
Prep Time: *10* Minutes
Cook Time: *3* Minutes
Total Time: *40* Minutes

INGREDIENTS

- 1 ½ tsp vinegar
- ½ tbs butter
- Salt
- Pepper
- 1 lb asparagus
- ¼ cup mint leaves
- 4 ounces radishes
- 1 tbs oil

DIRECTIONS

1. Cut the asparagus into pieces.
2. Cook the asparagus for 3 minutes in the butter.
3. Slice the radishes and toss with the asparagus in a bowl.
4. Mix the oil and the vinegar and pour the mixture over the vegetables.
5. Season with salt and pepper.
6. Slice the mint and toss with the vegetables, serve cold.

GINGER, BUTTERNUT SQUASH & SWEET POTATO

Serves: *8*
Prep Time: *20* Minutes
Cook Time: *1h 30* Minutes
Total Time: *2h 50* Minutes

INGREDIENTS

- 1 ginger
- 4 sweet potatoes
- 5 tbs oil
- 1 tbs salt
- 1 butternut squash
- 1 tbs pepper
- 3 onions

DIRECTIONS

1. Preheat the oven to 400F.
2. Cut the butternut squash and sweet potatoes.
3. Combine the squash, sweet potatoes, onions, ginger, oil, salt, and pepper.
4. Mix the ingredients together.

5. Bake for 40 minutes, then reduce the heat and cook for another 1 ½ hours.
6. Reduce the heat again and cook for another hour.
7. Serve warm.

BREADED TURKEY

Serves: **4**

Prep Time: **10** Minutes

Cook Time: **10** Minutes

Total Time: **20** Minutes

INGREDIENTS

- Bread crumbs
- Oil
- 4 turkey breasts
- Flour
- 3 eggs

DIRECTIONS

1. Dip the breasts into the flour, whisked eggs and bread crumbs in this order.
2. Fry in the oil until golden.
3. Serve with a salad.

LENTILS

Serves: **8**
Prep Time: ***12h 15*** Minutes
Cook Time: ***30*** Minutes
Total Time: ***12h 45*** Minutes

INGREDIENTS

- 5 ounces lentils
- Bay leaf
- 5 tomatoes
- Parsley
- 1 onion
- ½ cup celery
- 1 clove garlic
- Salt

- Pepper
- 1 carrot

DIRECTIONS

1. Soak the lentils for 12 hours.
2. Cook the onion, carrot, celery and garlic in a pot until the onion is ready.
3. Season with salt and pepper.
4. Add the tomatoes and cook until they become a sauce.
5. Add the lentils and cook until soft.
6. Serve sprinkled with parsley.

HUMMUS

Serves: 8
Prep Time: 20 Minutes
Cook Time: 0 Minutes
Total Time: 20 Minutes

INGREDIENTS

- 250g chickpeas

- 3 cloves garlic
- 1 tbs tahini
- Salt
- Pepper
- 1 lemon juice
- Oil

DIRECTIONS

1. Wash the chickpeas.
2. Place the ingredients in a blender and pulse, drizzling oil from time to time.

BEANS BURGERS

Serves: **2**

Prep Time: **10** Minutes

Cook Time: **10** Minutes

Total Time: **20** Minutes

INGREDIENTS

- 1 tin red kidney beans

- Parsley
- 1 clove garlic
- 1 chili pepper
- Salt
- Pepper

DIRECTIONS

1. Wash the beans, then combine with the chopped chili, garlic, parsley and the fried onion.
2. Season then form patties from the mixture.
3. Fry and serve with salad.

BORLOTTI BEAN

Serves: **4**

Prep Time: **10** Minutes

Cook Time: **30** Minutes

Total Time: **40** Minutes

INGREDIENTS

- 1 tin beans

- 1 clove garlic
- Salt
- Pepper
- Zucchini
- 1 egg
- Bread crumbs

DIRECTIONS

1. Crush the washed beans with oil, salt, pepper and garlic.
2. Fry the zucchini and dice.
3. Add the zucchini to the bean mixture.
4. Form long shaped fritters.
5. Roll in the whisked egg and then in the bread crumbs.
6. Fry in oil until golden.

FOIL COOKED FISH

Serves: **4**

Prep Time: **10** Minutes

Cook Time: **15** Minutes

Total Time: **25** Minutes

INGREDIENTS

- 1 fish
- Thyme
- Oil
- Salt
- Pepper

DIRECTIONS

1. Place the fish in a piece of foil.
2. Add thyme, oil, salt and pepper.
3. Close the foil around the fish.
4. Cook for 15 minutes at 190F.
5. Serve immediately.

GARLIC MUSHROOMS

Serves: 2

Prep Time: 5 Minutes

Cook Time: 5 Minutes

Total Time: 10 Minutes

INGREDIENTS

- 150g mushrooms
- Oil
- Salt
- Pepper
- 2 cloves garlic
- Parsley

DIRECTIONS

1. Wash the mushrooms and place in a frying pan with oil, salt, and pepper.
2. Once nearly cooked, add the garlic and cook for a few minutes.
3. Remove from heat and add parsley.
4. Serve immediately.

TOFU BURGER

Serves: **8**

Prep Time: **10** Minutes

Cook Time: **10** Minutes

Total Time: **20** Minutes

INGREDIENTS

- 9 ounces vegetables
- 1 clove garlic
- Salt
- Pepper
- 1 egg
- Tofu
- Cumin
- Chili powder
- Paprika

DIRECTIONS

1. Cook the vegetable shreddings in a frying pan until soft.
2. Add the garlic, salt, and pepper.
3. Allow to cool.

4. Add 1 whisked egg, and the spices to the vegetables.
5. Mix well and form patties.
6. Fry until brown on both sides.
7. Fry the tofu slices.
8. Serve on a bun topped with the fried tofu.

SWEET POTATOES FRIES

Serves: **4**

Prep Time: **10** Minutes

Cook Time: **5** Minutes

Total Time: **15** Minutes

INGREDIENTS

- 1 sweet potato
- Salt
- Pepper
- Oil
- 1 clove garlic

DIRECTIONS

1. Cut the potato in your desired shape.
2. Soften in boiling water for 1 minute.
3. Pat dry and fry in a pan of oil and garlic.
4. Cook for 5 minutes, season and serve.

CHICKEN

Serves: **4**

Prep Time: **20** Minutes

Cook Time: **50** Minutes

Total Time: **70** Minutes

INGREDIENTS

- 1 chicken
- Oil
- 1 clove garlic
- Zucchini
- Tomatoes
- Aubergine
- Salt
- Pepper

- Thyme

DIRECTIONS

1. Dress the chicken with oil, garlic, thyme, salt, and pepper.
2. Roast for 35 minutes at 190F.
3. Cut the vegetables into cubes, dress with oil and seasoning and roast for 20 minutes.
4. Serve the chicken with the vegetables.

SNACKS & DESSERTS

BLUEBERRY BAKED OATMEAL

Serves: **8**

Prep Time: **10** Minutes

Cook Time: **40** Minutes

Total Time: **50** Minutes

INGREDIENTS

- 1 cup rolled-oats
- ¼ cup chopped walnuts
- ¾ tsp ground cumin
- Salt
- ¼ cup maple syrup
- 1 ½ tsp vanilla
- 3 bananas
- 1 cup blueberries
- 1 cup milk
- 1 egg
- 2 tbs butter
- ½ tsp baking powder

DIRECTIONS

1. Preheat the oven to 375F.
2. Mix the oats, baking powder, half of the walnuts, cinnamon, and salt in a bowl.
3. In a cup mix the syrup, egg, milk, vanilla, and butter.
4. Spread the sliced banana into a greased pan.
5. Top with half of the berries and the oats.
6. Pour the wet ingredients over.
7. Sprinkle the remaining nuts and berries over.
8. Bake for 40 minutes.
9. Allow to cool for 10 minutes, then serve.

OATMEAL COOKIE GRANOLA

Serves: **12**
Prep Time: **10** Minutes
Cook Time: **30** Minutes
Total Time: **40** Minutes

INGREDIENTS

- 2 ¼ cups rolled oats

- ½ cup dried cranberries
- ½ cup chia seeds
- 1 tbs sugar
- ½ cup honey
- 4 tbs coconut oil
- 2 ½ tsp vanilla
- ½ cup chocolate chips
- 1 ½ tsp cinnamon
- 1 cup sliced almonds
- 1 tsp salt

DIRECTIONS

1. Preheat the oven to 325F.
2. Whisk the sugar, cinnamon, oats, chia seeds, salt, and almonds in a bowl.
3. In a pot combine the coconut oil, honey and vanilla and bring to a simmer.
4. Pour the mixture over the oats and coat well.
5. Bake for 30 minutes, tossing every 10 minutes.
6. Allow to cool for 5 minutes, then toss in the chocolate chips and the cranberries, serve cold.

HONEY WALNUTS

Serves: **4**

Prep Time: **5** Minutes

Cook Time: **15** Minutes

Total Time: **20** Minutes

INGREDIENTS

- walnuts
- honey
- cinnamon

DIRECTIONS
1. **Spread the nuts on a lined baking tray.**
2. **Cover with honey.**
3. **Bake for 15 minutes, dust cinnamon over.**

MUG CAKE

Serves: **2**

Prep Time: **5** Minutes

Cook Time: **2** Minutes

Total Time: 7 Minutes

INGREDIENTS

- 3 tbs monk fruit
- 1 egg white
- 1 tbs tapioca flour
- Salt
- 3 tbs chocolate chips
- 3 tbs butter
- 2 tbs cocoa powder
- ¼ tsp baking powder
- 1 tsp vanilla
- 2 tbs almond flour

DIRECTIONS

1. Melt the butter.
2. Mix the dry ingredients well.
3. Add the remaining ingredients and stir well.
4. Microwave for 90 seconds, serve immediately.

LEMON BITES

Serves: **4**

Prep Time: **10** Minutes

Cook Time: **40** Minutes

Total Time: **50** Minutes

INGREDIENTS
Crust
- 1 cup tapioca flour
- ½ cup monk fruit
- ¾ almond flour
- 1 stick grass fed butter
- ¼ tsp vanilla

Lemon filling
- ½ cup monk fruit
- 4 eggs
- 3 lemons
- ¼ cup flour

DIRECTIONS

1. Preheat the oven to 350F.
2. Mix all of the crust ingredients and press down in a dish.
3. Cook for 10 minutes.
4. Zest one lemon and juice them all in a bowl.
5. Add the filling ingredients.

6. Spread the filling over the crust and bake for 20 minutes, refrigerate, then serve.

CHIA PUDDING

Serves: 4
Prep Time: 5 Minutes
Cook Time: 0 Minutes
Total Time: 5 Minutes

INGREDIENTS

- 1 tsp vanilla
- 4 tbs chia seeds
- 2 tsp maple syrup
- 1 cup coconut milk
- ½ tsp maca powder

DIRECTIONS

1. Mix all of the ingredients in a bowl.
2. Refrigerate and serve with your desired toppings.

AVOCADO CAKE

Serves: **8**
Prep Time: **10** Minutes
Cook Time: **20** Minutes
Total Time: **30** Minutes

INGREDIENTS

- 1 tsp baking powder
- 2 tsp vanilla
- 3 tbs butter
- ¾ coconut milk
- ½ cup coconut flour
- ¼ cup tapioca flour
- ¼ cup almond flour
- 1 avocado
- 5 tbs cocoa powder
- ¾ cup munk fruit
- 2 tbs maple syrup
- 1 tbs yogurt
- 2 eggs

DIRECTIONS

1. Preheat the oven to 350F.
2. Mix the dry ingredients in a bowl.
3. Puree the avocado.
4. Mix the wet ingredients in another bowl.
5. Mix the wet and dry ingredients together.
6. Bake in a greased pan for 20 minutes.
7. Serve.

APPLE COOKIES

Serves: **8**
Prep Time: **10** Minutes
Cook Time: **15** Minutes
Total Time: **25** Minutes

INGREDIENTS

- 1 bag apple rings
- 1 can coconut milk
- ½ tbs coconut oil

- 3 tbs coconut
- ¼ cup honey
- ¼ cup chocolate chips
- 1 tbs butter
- 2 tsp vanilla
- Salt
- ¾ cup coconut sugar

DIRECTIONS

1. Mix the coconut milk, coconut oil, coconut sugar, vanilla, ½ tbs butter, honey, and salt in a saucepan.
2. Bring to a boil, then simmer for 10 minutes.
3. Refrigerate for at least an hour.
4. Remove from the fridge and stir in the coconut.
5. Spread the mixture over the apple rings.
6. Melt the chocolate chips and butter and drizzle over.

PUMPKIN CHEESECAKE BARS

Serves: **12**
Prep Time: **3** Hours

Cook Time: **40** Minutes

Total Time: **3h 40** Minutes

INGREDIENTS

- 1 ¾ cups graham cracker crumbs
- 15 ounces pumpkin puree
- ½ cup brown sugar
- ½ cup milk
- 8 ounces cream cheese
- 1 1/3 cups xylitol
- 4 eggs
- 1 egg white
- ½ tsp salt
- 1 tsp cinnamon
- Gelatin
- ½ cup butter
- ¼ cup cold water

Graham Cracker Crumbs

- 1 tsp cinnamon
- 1 tbs xylitol
- 4 tbs butter
- 1 ½ cup almond flour
- Salt

DIRECTIONS

1. Mix 4 tbs of melted butter, 1 tbs xylitol, ½ cups almond flour, ½ tsp salt, and 1 tsp cinnamon.
2. Press down the dough into a greased baking dish.
3. Beat the cream cheese and 1 1/3 cup xylitol until smooth.
4. Beat in 2 eggs
5. Pour over curst and bake at 350F for 20 minutes.
6. Mix ½ cup xylitol and 1 tbs molasses to create the brown sugar.
7. In a saucepan mix the yolks, pumpkin, the brown sugar, milk, salt, and cinnamon.
8. Cook for 10 minutes over low heat.
9. Pour the gelatin into cold water and allow to sit for 1 minute.
10. Heat and stir until the gelatin is dissolved, then stir into the pumpkin mixture.
11. Mix the egg white with 1 tbs of xylitol and beat for 5 minutes while on low heat.
12. Remove from heat and pour into the pumpkin mixture.
13. Spread over the cream cheese layer, cover and refrigerate for 3 hours.
14. Serve topped with whip cream.

PUMPKIN CHEESECAKE

Serves: **8**

Prep Time: **10** Minutes

Cook Time: **0** Minutes

Total Time: **10** Minutes

INGREDIENTS
Crust
- 4 tbs butter
- 1 tsp chia seeds
- 2 tbs honey
- 1 ½ cup almond flour
- 1 tsp almond milk
- Cinnamon

Filling
- 1 15-ounces can pumpkin puree
- Whip cream
- 1 tsp pumpkin spice
- 8 ounces whipped cream cheese
- ½ tsp nutmeg
- Cinnamon
- 1/3 cup xylitol
- 1/3 tbs maple syrup

DIRECTIONS

1. Blend all of the crust ingredients and pat down into a pie dish.
2. Blend all of the filling ingredients.

3. Place the filling on top of the crust.
4. Chill for at least 1 hour, then serve.

CELERY CARROT JUICE

Serves: 1
Prep Time: 5 Minutes
Cook Time: 0 Minutes
Total Time: 5 Minutes

INGREDIENTS

- ½ beet
- 1 celery stick
- 1 carrot
- 3 parsley

DIRECTIONS

1. Blend all of the ingredients together.
2. Serve immediately.

SPINACH SMOOTHIE

Serves: *1*
Prep Time: *5* Minutes
Cook Time: *0* Minutes
Total Time: *5* Minutes

INGREDIENTS

- Almond milk
- 1 banana
- Handful of blueberries
- 1 cup spinach
- 5 peach slices
- Handful of walnuts

DIRECTIONS

1. **Blend all of the ingredients together.**
2. **Serve immediately.**

KALE SMOOTHIE

Serves: 1
Prep Time: 5 Minutes
Cook Time: 0 Minutes
Total Time: 5 Minutes

INGREDIENTS

- Coconut water
- Water
- ½ banana
- 4 strawberries
- 3 kale laves
- 3 dates
- 1 tsp peanut butter
- ½ avocado
- 1 cup spinach

DIRECTIONS

1. Blend all of the ingredients together.
2. Serve immediately.

STRAWBERRIES SMOOTHIE

Serves: **1**

Prep Time: **5** Minutes

Cook Time: **0** Minutes

Total Time: **5** Minutes

INGREDIENTS

- Banana
- Parsley
- Strawberries
- Almonds
- Flaxseeds
- Spinach
- Coconut water
- Blackberries

DIRECTIONS

1. **Blend all of the ingredients together.**
2. **Serve immediately.**

PINEAPPLE SMOOTHIE

Serves: **1**

Prep Time: **5** Minutes

Cook Time: **0** Minutes

Total Time: **5** Minutes

INGREDIENTS

- Butterhead lettuce
- Coconut flakes
- Water
- Pineapple
- Watermelon
- Banana
- Pomegranate seeds
- Flaxseeds

DIRECTIONS

1. Blend all of the ingredients together.
2. Serve immediately.

MANGO SALSA JUICE

Serves: *1*
Prep Time: 5 Minutes
Cook Time: *0* Minutes
Total Time: 5 Minutes

INGREDIENTS

- 1 mango
- ½ lime
- ¼ yellow pepper
- ½ Jalapeno pepper
- 1/3 cucumber
- 2 green onions
- ¼ cup cilantro

DIRECTIONS

1. Peel the mango and cut.
2. Blend all of the ingredients together.
3. Serve immediately.

GINGER JUICE

Serves: 1
Prep Time: 5 Minutes
Cook Time: 0 Minutes
Total Time: 5 Minutes

INGREDIENTS

- ½-inch ginger root
- 2 ribs of celery
- 3 kale leaves
- ½ small pineapple

DIRECTIONS

1. Blend all of the ingredients together.
2. Serve immediately.

OATS SMOOTHIE

Serves: *1*
Prep Time: *5* Minutes
Cook Time: *0* Minutes
Total Time: *5* Minutes

INGREDIENTS

- Oats
- Honey
- Orange juice
- Blueberries
- Banana
- Raspberries
- Mango

DIRECTIONS

1. **Blend all of the ingredients together.**
2. **Serve immediately.**

KIWI JUICE

Serves: *1*

Prep Time: *5* Minutes

Cook Time: *0* Minutes

Total Time: *5* Minutes

INGREDIENTS

- Kiwi
- Pomegranate

DIRECTIONS

1. **Skin the kiwis.**
2. **Scoop out the pomegranate seeds.**
3. **Blend them together.**
4. **Serve immediately.**

PAIN KILLER JUICE

Serves: **1**

Prep Time: **5** Minutes

Cook Time: **0** Minutes

Total Time: **5** Minutes

INGREDIENTS

- A handful of cilantro
- Ginger
- 2 ribs celery
- ½ pineapple
- 1 head Romaine lettuce

DIRECTIONS

1. **Blend all of the ingredients together.**
2. **Serve immediately.**

THANK YOU FOR READING THIS BOOK!

Made in the USA
Middletown, DE
30 April 2019